FREE FROM ADHD:
A positive guide to be free from ADHD

Robert j. Chatier

Table of contents

Chapter 1

Overview of ADHD
Attention deficit hyperactivity disorder (ADHD) is a condition that affects people's behaviors. People with ADHD might look restless, may have difficulties focusing, and may act on impulse.

Symptoms of ADHD tend to be detected at an early age and may become more obvious as a child's circumstances change, such as when they start school.

Most instances are diagnosed when children are 3 to 7 years old, however, occasionally it's detected later in childhood.

Sometimes ADHD was not noticed while someone was a kid, and they are diagnosed later as an adult.

The symptoms of ADHD normally improve with age, but many individuals who were diagnosed with the illness at a young age continue to encounter challenges.

People with ADHD may also have other issues, such as sleep and anxiety disorders.

Getting assistance
Many youngsters go through times when they're restless or inattentive. This is frequently entirely natural and does not necessarily suggest they have ADHD.

But you should address your concerns with your child's teacher, their school's special educational needs coordinator (SENCO), or a GP if you suspect their conduct may be unusual for most children their age.

It's also a good idea to go to a GP if you're an adult and suspect you may have ADHD but were not diagnosed with the disease as a kid.

What causes attention deficit hyperactivity disorder (ADHD)?
The specific etiology of ADHD is unclear, however, the disorder has been demonstrated to run in families.

Research has also discovered several probable changes in the brains of persons with ADHD when compared with those without the illness.

Other variables indicated as possibly having a function in ADHD include:

being born early (before the 37th week of pregnancy) (before the 37th week of pregnancy)
having a low birth weight\smoking or alcohol or drug addiction during pregnancy
ADHD may occur in persons of any intellectual level, however, it's more frequent in those with learning disabilities.

How attention deficit hyperactivity disorder (ADHD) is handled

For children with ADHD, while there's no cure, it may be controlled with proper educational assistance, guidance, support for parents and affected children, and medication, if required.

For adults with ADHD, medication is frequently the primary treatment administered, but psychological treatments such as cognitive behavioral therapy (CBT) may also assist.

Living with attention deficit hyperactivity disorder (ADHD) (ADHD)

Parents of children with ADHD

Looking for a kid with ADHD may be tough, but it's vital to remember that they cannot change their behaviors.

Some day-to-day tasks could be more challenging for you and your kid, including:

getting your kid to sleep at night
getting ready for school on time
listening to and following out instructions\being organized\social gatherings
shopping
Adults with ADHD
Adults with ADHD may discover they have difficulty with:

organization and time management\following directions
focused and finishing tasks
dealing with stress\feeling restless or impatient\impulsiveness and risk-taking
Some individuals may also have difficulty with relationships or social engagement.

Chapter 2

Symptoms of attention deficit hyperactivity disorder (ADHD) (ADHD)
The symptoms of attention deficit hyperactivity disorder (ADHD) may be divided into 2 categories of behavioral problems:

inattentiveness (difficulty concentrating and concentration) (difficulty concentrating and focusing)
hyperactivity and impulsiveness
Many persons with ADHD have challenges that fit into both these categories, although this is not always the case.

For example, roughly 2 to 3 in 10 persons with the disorder have difficulty with concentrating and concentration, but not with hyperactivity or impulsiveness.

This kind of ADHD is also known as attention deficit disorder (ADD) (ADD). ADD may often go unrecognized since the symptoms may be less visible.

ADHD is more typically diagnosed in males than in girls. Girls are more likely to exhibit signs of inattentiveness exclusively and are less likely to demonstrate disruptive activity that makes ADHD symptoms more visible. This implies females who have ADHD may not always be diagnosed.

Symptoms in children and teens
The signs of ADHD in children and teens are established, and they're frequently visible before the age of 6. They occur in more than 1 setting, such as at home and school.

Children may show indications of both inattentiveness and hyperactivity and impulsiveness, or they may have evidence of only 1 of these kinds of behavior.

Inattentiveness (difficulty concentrating and concentration) (difficulty concentrating and focusing)
The major indications of inattentiveness are:

having a short attention span and being quickly distracted\smacking thoughtless errors – for example, in schoolwork\disappearing forgetful or forgetting things\being unable to stick to boring jobs or time-consuming\appearing to be unable to listen to or follow instructions continually shifting activity or task\having difficulties coordinating activities
Hyperactivity and impulsiveness
The primary indications of hyperactivity and impulsiveness are:

being unable to remain motionless, particularly in peaceful or quiet situations continually fidgeting\being unable to focus on activities excessive physical movement\excessive talking

being unable to wait for their turn\acting without thinking\interrupting talks

little or no sensation of risk

These symptoms may create considerable issues in a child's life, such as underachievement at school, poor social contact with other children and adults, and difficulty with discipline.

Related problems in children and teens with ADHD

Although not usually the case, some children may also exhibit evidence of other issues or conditions with ADHD, such as:

anxiety disorder - which causes your kid to worry and be tense most of the time; it may also create physical symptoms, such as a fast heartbeat, perspiration, and dizziness

oppositional defiant disorder (ODD) - This is characterized by negative and disruptive

behaviors, especially towards authority figures, such as parents and teachers
conduct disorder - this generally comprises a predisposition towards severely antisocial activities, such as stealing, fighting, vandalism, and injuring people or animals
depression
sleep issues - finding it difficult to go to sleep at night, and having inconsistent sleeping patterns
autism spectrum disorder (ASD) - this impairs social interaction, communication, interests, and conduct
dyspraxia — a disorder that inhibits physical coordination
epilepsy - an illness that affects the brain and produces recurring fits or seizures
Tourette's syndrome — a disorder of the nervous system, defined by a mix of uncontrollable noises and movements (tics) (tics)
learning issues – such as dyslexia
Symptoms in adults

In adults, the symptoms of ADHD are more difficult to characterize. This is primarily owing to a paucity of studies on people with ADHD.

As ADHD is a developmental illness, it's thought it cannot develop in adults without it initially presenting during infancy. But symptoms of ADHD in adolescents and teens typically remain until maturity.

How inattentiveness, hyperactivity, and impulsiveness impact adults may be extremely different from the way they influence youngsters.

For example, hyperactivity tends to lessen in adults, whereas inattentiveness tends to stay as the stresses of adult life mount.

Adult signs of ADHD also tend to be significantly more modest than childhood symptoms.

Some professionals have proposed the following as a list of symptoms related to ADHD in adults:

carelessness and lack of attention to detail
continuously beginning new activities before completing old ones
weak organizing skills
inability to concentrate or prioritize
repeatedly missing or misplacing stuff
forgetfulness
restlessness and edginess\difficulty keeping quiet, and speaking out of turn\blurting out responses and often interrupting others\mood swings, irritability and a quick temper\inability to deal with stress\extreme impatience\taking risks in activities, often with little or no regard for personal safety or the safety of others – for example, driving dangerously
Related conditions in adults with ADHD
As with ADHD in children and teens, ADHD in adults may occur with various linked issues or conditions.

One of the most frequent is depression. Other conditions that adults may have alongside ADHD include:

personality disorders — situations in which an individual varies markedly from the ordinary person in terms of how they think, perceive, feel or connect to others
bipolar disorder – a condition affecting your mood, which may swing from one extreme to another\obsessive compulsive disorder (OCD) – is a condition that produces obsessive thoughts and compulsive conduct
The behavioral disorders linked with ADHD may also produce problems such as difficulty with relationships and social engagement.

Chapter 3

Causes of ADHD
The specific etiology of attention deficit hyperactivity disorder (ADHD) is not entirely known, however a mix of variables is likely to be involved.

Genetics\ADHD tends to run in families and, in most instances, it's assumed the genes you get from your parents play a crucial component in developing the disorder.

Research reveals that parents and siblings of someone with ADHD are more likely to develop ADHD themselves.

However, the method ADHD is inherited is likely to be complicated and is not assumed to be tied to a single genetic flaw.

Brain function and structure
Research has revealed a number of probable variations in the brains of persons with ADHD from those without the illness, however the precise importance of these is not apparent.

For example, research employing brain scans have revealed that specific parts of the brain may be smaller in persons with ADHD, whilst other areas may be bigger.

Other research have shown that patients with ADHD may have an imbalance in the quantity of neurotransmitters in the brain, or that these chemicals may not operate effectively.

Groups at risk
Certain persons are also regarded to be more at risk of ADHD, such as:

who were born prematurely (before the 37th week of pregnancy) or with a low birth weight\with epilepsy\with brain damage - which occurred either in the womb or after a serious head injury later in life.

Chapter 4

Treatment of ADHD
Treatment for attention deficit hyperactivity disorder (ADHD) may help ease the symptoms and make the condition much less of a concern in day-to-day living.

ADHD may be treated with medication or therapy, but a mix of both is frequently optimal.

Treatment is generally handled by a professional, such as a pediatrician or psychiatrist, but the condition may be managed by a GP.

Medicine
There are 5 kinds of medication authorized for the treatment of ADHD:

methylphenidate\lisdexamfetamine

dexamfetamine

atomoxetine\guanfacine

These drugs are not a permanent solution for ADHD but may help someone with the disease focus better, be less impulsive, feel calmer, and acquire and practice new skills.

Other medications need to be taken every day, whereas some may be taken simply on school days. Treatment interruptions are sometimes indicated to examine if the drug is still required.

If you were not diagnosed with ADHD until adulthood, a GP and expert may explore which drugs and treatments are suited for you.

If you or your kid is prescribed one of these drugs, you'll usually be given tiny dosages at first, which may then be progressively raised. You or your kid will need to visit a GP for frequent check-ups to verify the therapy is functioning successfully and check for indications of any side effects or concerns.

It's crucial to let the GP know about any adverse effects and speak to them if you feel you need to stop or modify therapy.

Your doctor will explain how long you should take your therapy however, in many circumstances, medication is maintained for as long as it is helpful.

Methylphenidate
Methylphenidate is the most often used drug for ADHD. It belongs to a category of drugs called stimulants, which function by raising activity in the brain, especially in regions that play a role in regulating attention and conduct.

Methylphenidate may be provided to adults, teens, and children over the age of 5 with ADHD.

The drug may be taken as either immediate-release tablets (small amounts given 2 to 3 times a day) or as modified-release tablets (administered once a day in the morning, with the dosage delivered throughout the day) (taken once a day in the morning, with the dose released throughout the day).

Common side effects of methylphenidate include:

a modest rise in blood pressure and heart rate\lack of appetite, which might lead to weight loss or poor weight gain
difficulties sleeping\headaches
stomach aches\feeling angry, irritated, melancholy, apprehensive, or tense.

Lisdexamfetamine
Lisdexamfetamine is a medication that activates particular areas of the brain. It enhances concentration, helps concentrate

attention, and minimizes impulsive behaviors.

It may be provided to teens and children over the age of 5 with ADHD if at least 6 weeks of therapy with methylphenidate has not helped.

Adults may be administered lisdexamfetamine as the first-choice drug instead of methylphenidate.

Lisdexamfetamine comes in capsule form, used once a day.

Common side effects of lisdexamfetamine include:

reduced appetite, which might lead to weight loss or poor weight gain
aggression\drowsiness
dizziness
headaches
diarrhea

nausea and vomiting
Dexamfetamine
Dexamfetamine is comparable to lisdexamfetamine and functions in the same manner. It may be provided to adults, teens, and children over the age of 5 with ADHD.

Dexamfetamine is normally used as a pill 2 to 4 times a day, however, an oral solution is also available.

Common side effects of dexamphetamine include:

reduced appetite
mood swings
agitation and aggression
dizziness\headaches
diarrhea\nausea and vomiting
Atomoxetine
Atomoxetine acts differently from other ADHD drugs.

It's a selective noradrenaline reuptake inhibitor (SNRI), which means it raises the quantity of a chemical in the brain called noradrenaline.This molecule delivers information between brain cells, and boosting it may assist attention and help regulate impulses.

Atomoxetine may be administered to adults, teens, and children over the age of 5 if it's not feasible to utilize methylphenidate or lisdexamfetamine. It's also permitted for usage in adults if signs of ADHD are proven.

Atomoxetine comes in pill form, commonly taken once or twice a day.

Common side effects of atomoxetine include:

a modest rise in blood pressure and heart rate

nausea and vomiting\stomach aches\trouble sleeping\dizziness\headaches\irritability Atomoxetine has also been related to certain more significant side effects that are crucial to watch out for, including suicidal thoughts and liver damage.

If either you or your kid starts to feel sad or suicidal while taking this prescription, talk to your doctor.

Guanfacine
Guanfacine operates on an area of the brain to promote attention, and it also regulates blood pressure.

It may be administered to teens and children above the age of 5 if it's not feasible to utilize methylphenidate or lisdexamfetamine. Guanfacine should not be provided to adults with ADHD.

Guanfacine is commonly taken as a pill once a day, in the morning or evening.

Common side effects include:

weariness or fatigue
headache\abdominal pain
dry mouth
Therapy
As well as taking medication, several treatments may be effective in treating ADHD in children, teens, and adults. Therapy is often beneficial in addressing related issues, such as behavior or anxiety disorders, that may occur with ADHD.Here are some of the treatments that may be employed.

Psychoeducation
Psychoeducation means you or your kid will be encouraged to address ADHD and its implications. It may assist children, teens and adults make sense of being diagnosed

with ADHD and can allow you to deal and live with the disease.

Behavior therapy
Behavior therapy offers help for caretakers of children with ADHD and may include teachers as well as parents. Behavior treatment generally comprises behavior management, which employs a system of incentives to help your kid to attempt to control their ADHD.

If your kid has ADHD, you may select the sorts of behaviors you wish to promote, such as sitting at the table to eat. Your youngster is then given some form of little incentive for excellent conduct.

For instructors, behavior management entails understanding how to design and organize activities, and praise and encourage children for even very tiny amounts of development.

Parent training and education courses
If your kid has ADHD, carefully specialized parent training and education courses may help you learn particular methods of communicating with your child, and playing and working with them to improve their attention and conduct.

You may also be provided parent training before your kid is officially diagnosed with ADHD.

These sessions are normally organized in groups of roughly 10 to 12 parents. A course normally comprises 10 to 16 sessions, lasting up to 2 hours each.

Being given a parent training and education course does not indicate you have been a terrible parent - it attempts to educate parents and caregivers about behavior management while improving confidence in your abilities to assist your kid and enhance your connection.

Social skills training
Social skills training includes your kid taking part in role-play settings and seeks to educate them on how to act in social circumstances by understanding how their conduct affects others.

Cognitive behavioral treatment (CBT) (CBT) CBT is a talking treatment that may help you manage your difficulties by altering the way you think and conduct. A therapist would aim to influence how you or your kid feels about a problem, which might in turn possibly affect their behaviors.

CBT may be carried out with a therapist alone or in a group.

Other possible therapies
There are other methods of treating ADHD that some individuals with the illness find beneficial, such as cutting out particular foods and taking vitamins. However, there's

no solid proof they work, and they should not be tried without medical counsel.

Diet

People with ADHD should eat a healthy, balanced diet. Do not cut off foods before obtaining medical advice.

Some individuals may discover a correlation between kinds of food and exacerbating ADHD symptoms. If this is the case, maintain a journal of everything you eat and drink, and what conduct follows. Discuss this with a GP, who may recommend you to a dietician (a healthcare practitioner who specializes in nutrition) (a healthcare professional who specializes in nutrition).Supplements\Some research has shown that supplements of omega-3 and omega-6 fatty acids may be useful for persons with ADHD, however, the data supporting this is relatively limited.

It's advised to speak to a GP before taking any supplements since some might mix adversely with medication or make it less effective.

You should also note that certain supplements should not be used long-term, since they might reach harmful amounts in your body.

Tips for Parents
If you're the parent of a kid with ADHD:

be sure your GP or specialist helps you understand the difference between ADHD and any other problems your child may have\think about who else needs to know about your child's ADHD, such as their school or nursery\find out the side effects of any medicine your child takes and what you need to look out for\getting to know people at local support groups can stop you feeling isolated and help you to cope.

Chapter 5

Living with attention deficit hyperactivity disorder (ADHD) may be stressful since the symptoms can make ordinary tasks more of a strain.

It's crucial to acquire the help you need to understand and deal with your or your child's illness.

Ways to cope for parents of children with ADHD
Caring for a kid with attention deficit hyperactivity disorder (ADHD) may be tough. The impulsive, bold, and disorganized actions characteristic of ADHD may make routine tasks tedious and distressing.

Although it might be tough at times, it's crucial to remember that a kid with ADHD cannot alter their actions. People with

ADHD might find it difficult to inhibit impulses, which means they may not pause to examine a situation or the repercussions before they act.

If you're caring for a youngster with ADHD, you may find this information useful.

Plan the day
Plan the day so your youngster understands what to anticipate. Set routines may make a difference in how a youngster with ADHD copes with regular life.

For example, if your kid needs to get ready for school, break it down into organized phases, so they know precisely what they need to do.

Set clear limits
Make sure everyone understands what conduct is expected, and encourage good behavior with prompt praise or awards. Be unambiguous, utilizing enforced

consequences, such as taking away a privilege, if limits are overstepped, and follow them through consistently.

Be positive
Give particular appreciation. Instead of stating a general: "Thanks for doing that," you may say: "You cleaned the dishes exceptionally well. Thank you."

This will make it plain to your youngster that you're delighted and why.

Giving directions
If you're asking your youngster to do anything, provide quick directions and be explicit. Instead of asking: "Can you clean your bedroom?" say: "Please put your toys into the box and put the books back onto the shelf."

This makes it apparent what your kid has to accomplish and allows praise when they do it correctly.

Incentive scheme
Set up your incentive program using a points or star chart, so excellent conduct may earn a privilege. For example, behaving nicely on a shopping trip can earn your youngster time on the computer or some form of the game.

Involve your kid in it and enablethem to help select what the privileges will be.

These charts require frequent modifications otherwise they grow dull. Targets should be:

immediate – for example, daily\intermediate – for example, weekly\long-term – for example, 3-monthly Try to concentrate on only 1 or 2 behaviors at a time.

Intervene early
Watch for warning signals. If your youngster appears like they're growing irritated,

overstimulated, and ready to lose self-control, intervene.

Distract your youngster, if feasible, by pulling them away from the scenario. This may calm them down.

Social circumstances
Keep social encounters brief and sweet. Invite others to play, but keep playtimes brief so your youngster does not lose self-control. Do not seek to do this while your kid is feeling weary or hungry, such as after a day at school.

Exercise
Make sure your youngster receives plenty of physical movement throughout the day. Walking, skipping, and playing sports might assist your youngsters to tire themselves out and increase their quality of sleep.

Make sure they're not doing anything too rigorous or stimulating close to sleep.

Read our physical activity recommendations for children and young people, which contain advice on being active, and how much exercise you and your kid should be doing.

Eating
Keep an eye on what your youngster consumes. If your kid is hyperactive after eating specific foods, which may include additives or caffeine, maintain a journal of them and discuss them with a GP.

Bedtime
Stick to a regimen. Make sure your youngster goes to bed at the same time each night and gets up at the same time in the morning.

Avoid over stimulating activities in the hours before night, such as computer games or watching TV.

Night time
Sleep issues with ADHD may be a vicious spiral. ADHD may lead to sleep issues, which in turn can make symptoms worse.

Many youngsters with ADHD will continually get up after being put to bed and have disrupted sleep habits. Trying a sleep-friendly regimen may benefit your kid and make bedtime less of a conflict.

Help at school
Children with ADHD typically have issues with their conduct in school, and the illness may significantly impair a child's academic achievement.

Speak to your kid's teachers or their school's special educational needs coordinator (SENCO) about any additional help your child may require.

Adults with ADHD

If you're an adult living with ADHD, you may find the following suggestions useful:

if you find it hard to remain organized, then write lists, maintain diaries, post up reminders and set aside some time to plan what you need to accomplish
blow off steam by exercising frequently
discover techniques to assist you to relax, such as listening to music or practicing breathing exercises for stress\if you have a job, talk to your employer about your illness, and explore whatever they can do to assist you to work better\if you're in college or university, enquire about what adaptations may be made to accommodate you, such as more time to finish examinations and coursework
speak to a doctor about your eligibility to drive, since you'll need to inform the Driver and Vehicle Licensing Agency (DVLA) if your ADHD impacts your driving\contact or join a local or national support group —

these groups may bring you in contact with other individuals in a similar position, and can be a wonderful source of support, information, and assistance.